THE LIFE ROBBING PAIN OF TMD

WHY ME?

© Dr. Mac Lee 2021

This book is dedicated to Dr. Bernard Jankleson, father of neuromuscular dentistry.

- Over fifty years ago, Dr. Bernard Jankleson developed neuromuscular dentistry, an answer to your life robbing pain.

- In 1979, Dr. Jankleson founded the International College of Craniomandibular Orthopedics (ICCMO.org); ICCMO endorses this book.

- If you are like many TMD sufferers, you have been searching for a long time with no answers or help. Specially trained neuromuscular dentists have answers.

- This digital book is one of ICCMO's goals to spread the word of neuromuscular dentistry to the world.

TABLE OF CONTENTS

INTRODUCTION

If you have life robbing TMD pain, know that it is real, and you are not alone!

The purpose of this E book is to explain, in layman's terms, why you have this horrible condition and what can be done to get relief.

I have been studying this extremely confusing condition for over forty years. In the last ten years, I have at last started to understand TMD and have learned techniques to help those who suffer.

Disclaimer: The information in this book is not diagnostic, it is educational information about a very confusing but serious condition called TMD.

INTRODUCTION

T he book will cover the basic TMD symptoms of popping jaw joint, painful joint, head pain, and a combination of these life robbing problems.

The various symptoms are due in part to functional and structural relationships between the jaw joint, teeth, muscles, ligaments, tendons, fascia, and the individual's negative response to these relationships. Only specially trained dentists understand these relationships.

Because of the pain's location, people turn to medicine instead of the dental profession. As you will see, the mouth and all its parts can create the pain you are feeling.

CHAPTER ONE: WHAT IS TMD? WHY ME?

- Your pains are real! You are not imagining the pain and you are not alone. Millions and millions of people around the world are suffering as you are.

- TMD stands for Tempro Mandibular Disorder. It is also called TMJ. Yes, very confusing names that can be blamed on the dental profession.

- The condition is confusing because it is probably hard for you to understand as to why one person has pain, and another does not.

- It is confusing because Health Care Providers such as chiropractors, massage therapist, physical therapist, acupuncturists, myofunctional therapists, dentists, treat with variable outcomes.

- It is complicated because it involves teeth, jaws, jaw joints, tendons, ligaments, muscles, spinal cord, neck, shoulders, hips and feet. "The foot bone is connected to the head bone."

WHAT IS TMD? WHY ME?

- It is complicated because it can involve history of accidents, orthodontic treatment, hormones, emotions, etc.

- It is frustrating because family and friends don't understand your pain. If they believe your pain, they are frustrated because they don't know how to help!

- The ultimate frustration is to have an MRI or CAT Scan only to have the specialist say, "There is nothing wrong with YOU!"

- The focus of this TMD/TMJ book will be on people in pain!

- Knowing that YOUR pain is real and understanding this confusing, painful condition is the first step in healing!

WHAT IS TMD? WHY ME?

If you have had MRIs, CAT Scans, seen neurologists, ENT, chiropractors, massage therapists, dentists, etc and have not found relief, listen to these people who have been treated with neuromuscular principles:

- https://www.youtube.com/watch?v=eojeFP2CxIQ&t=38s

- https://www.youtube.com/watch?v=wTUyI-zqM3k

- https://www.youtube.com/watch?v=adXWPpYEp5k

- https://www.youtube.com/watch?v=HnvsdHnpKG0&t=3s

- https://www.youtube.com/watch?v=nF9G6RQEq74

- https://www.youtube.com/watch?v=umVcrS1Avzk

CHAPTER TWO: UNDERSTANDING YOUR TM JOINT

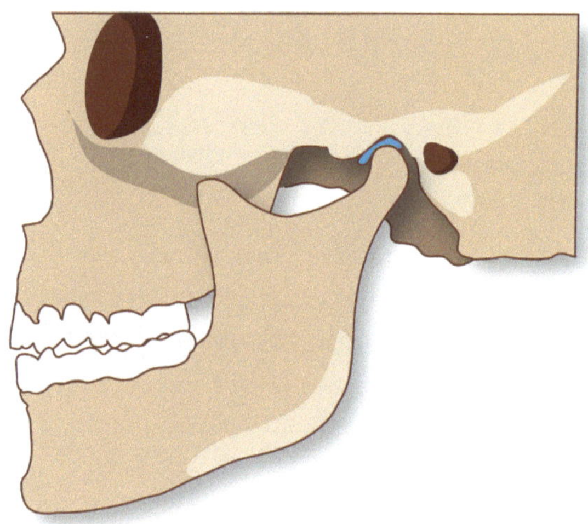

- The jaw joints are absolutely the most unique and fascinating joints in the body.

- Understanding where they are and how they work will help you understand your TMD pain.

- The jaw is capable of extremely complicated maneuvers and has responsibilities in eating, talking, swallowing, and breathing.

- This image will be used throughout the book and will illustrate what is normal and what is not.

UNDERSTANDING YOUR TM JOINT

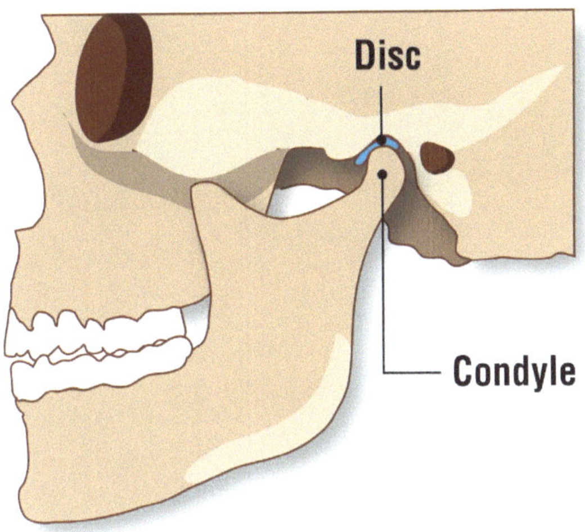

- The jaw is only connected to the skull by muscles, tendons, ligaments and skin all of which can generate pain.

- Their job is to hold the jaw in a balanced relationship to the skull as indicated in the illustration.

- To be normal, the joint (condyle) must sit in its socket with space to move around in.

- The joint has a "disc" that sits on top of the condyle to help it slide down the socket with ease.

- The disc is the blue life saver shaped object in the illustration.

- Keep your eyes on the blue disc; when it is not in the right location, bad things happen.

UNDERSTANDING YOUR TM JOINT

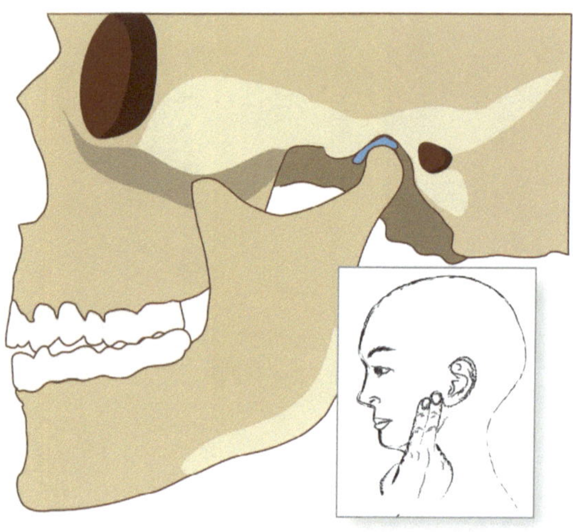

- You can feel your jaw joints by putting your fingers in front of both ear canals and open and close the jaw. What you are feeling is the condyle itself.
- Move the jaw forward and back.
- Now move left and right.
- You should start to appreciate the complexity of the joint.
- When the joint is not able to work correctly, bad things can happen.

CHAPTER THREE: POPPING AND NOISY JOINT SOUNDS

Normal Disc And Joint

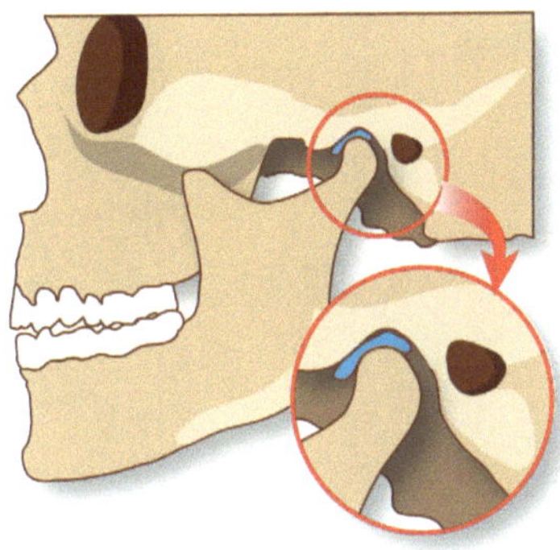

Disc "Popped" Off Condyle

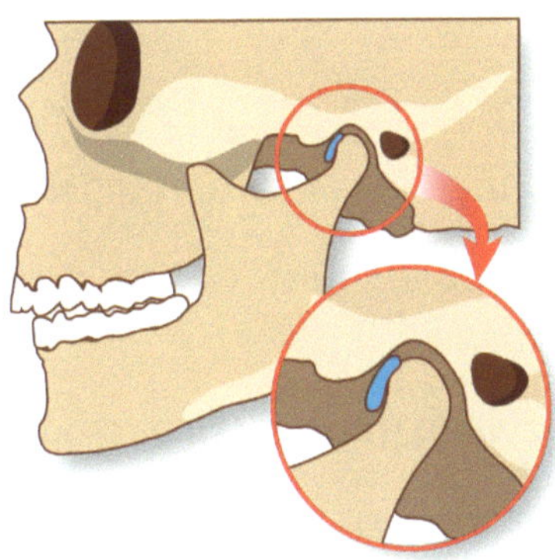

POPPING AND NOISY JOINT SOUNDS

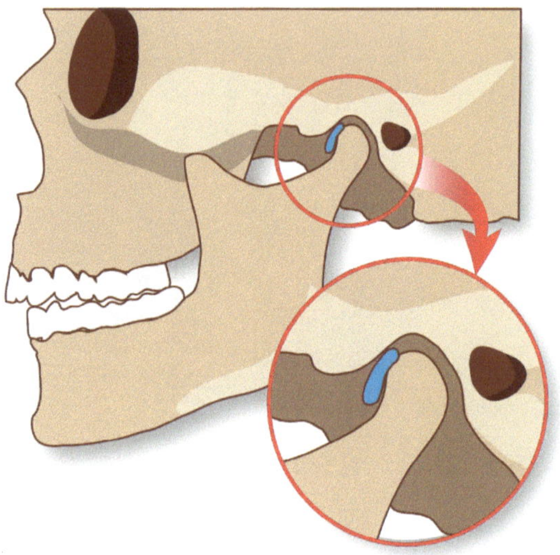

- A clicking joint is the sign of something wrong.

- The disc that is supposed to sit on top of the condyle, slides off and on the condyle.

- It makes a sound when popping in and out position.

- Most clicking joints are not painful.

- Over the years, this incorrect joint/disc relationship will only get worse.

OPENING AND CLOSING OF THE JAW CAUSES THE "POP!"

Blue Disc Is In Front Of Condyle

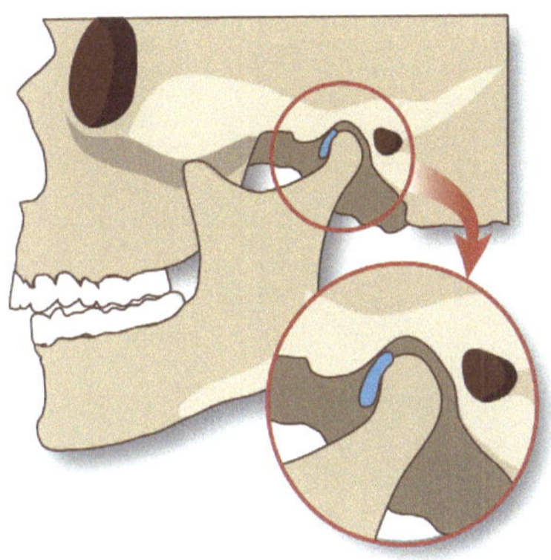

Blue Disc Pops Back On Condyle

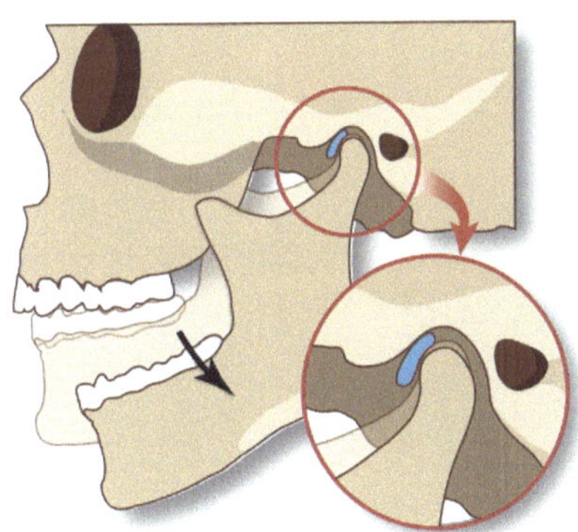

POPPING AND NOISY JOINT SOUNDS

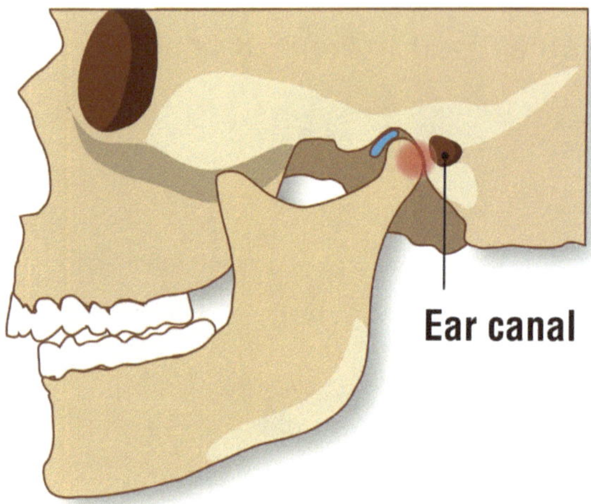

- The hole you see next to the joint is the ear canal.

- The bone is thin between the condyle and the ear canal.

- The pushing of condyle towards the ear complex can create feelings of stuffy ears, ear drainage and in some instances, ringing of the ears.

CHAPTER FOUR: PAIN IN THE JOINT/EAR AREA

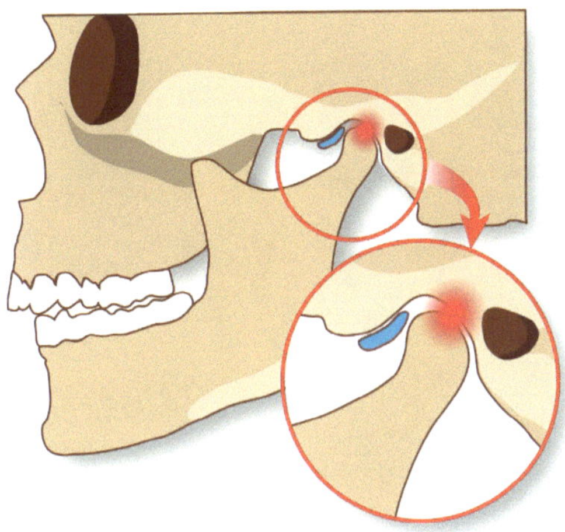

- There is a bundle of nerves and blood vessels behind the condyle. For those who like to research, the area is called the Retrodiscal pad.

- When the jaw and condyle are pushed back even further as demonstrated in the illustration, it pushes on this nerve complex (in red).

- When a nerve is being pushed, it responds with pain.

- For those of you with pain in the ear area, see if you relate to Kim's story:

    https://www.youtube.com/watch?v=adXWPpYEp5k

PAIN IN THE JOINT/EAR AREA

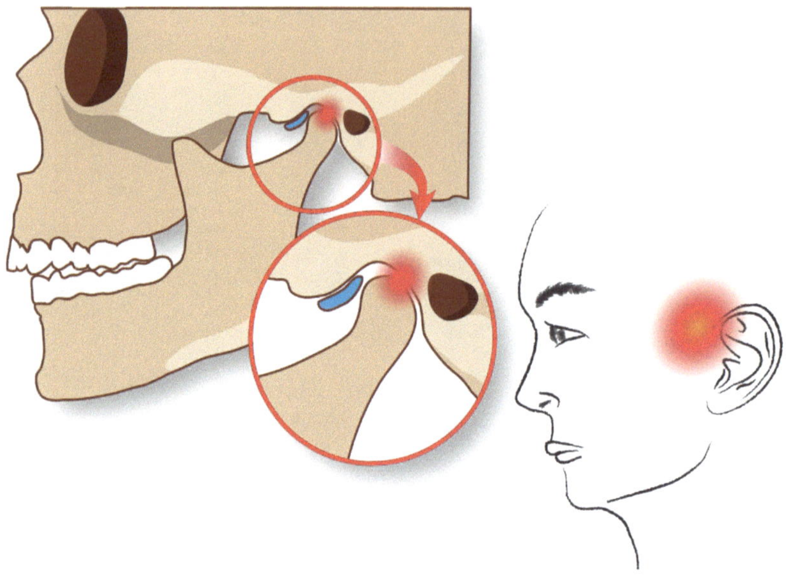

- If you went to the video, you could see how painful a joint like this can be.

- Sometimes the joint pain is confused with ear pain. However, you are told by MD, ENT, or Nurse Practitioner that there is nothing wrong with your ear.

- While TMD pain seems to be a medical problem, it may in fact be dental.

PAIN IN THE JOINT/EAR AREA

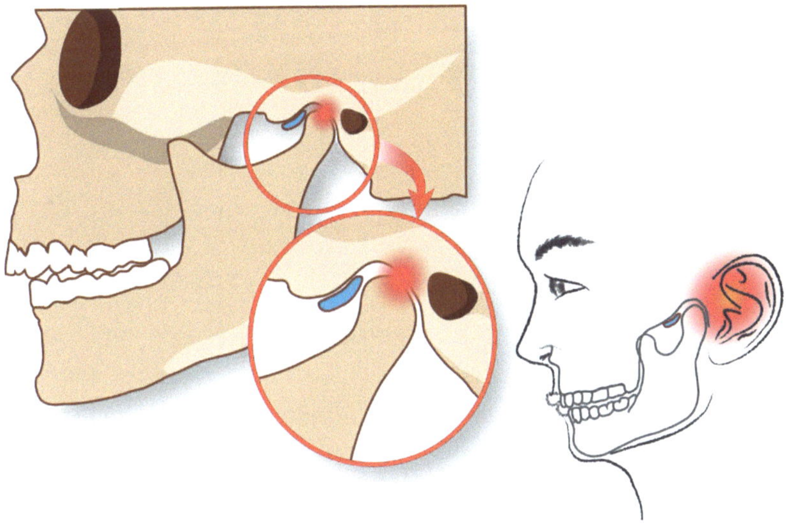

- The improper position of the condyle and disc causes a cascade of events that are painful and confusing.

- All the before mentioned ligaments, teeth, tendons and muscles have nerve innervations and can create pain when the jaw-to-jaw relationship is not correct.

- The reason why will be demonstrated later in the book.

WHY IS THE TM JOINT IN THE IMPROPER POSITION?

- The answer is complicated and disputed among dentists.

- The upper "Jaw" is part of the skull but for simplicity, I will use the term jaw-to-jaw relationship.

- When the jaw-to-jaw relationship is not correct, during closure, the lower jaw is pulled back so back teeth touch. This pushes the condyle back and squeezes the disc off the condyle.

- The distance it is pushed back dictates the joint damage/pain over time.

- Conservative treatment is to signal the brain that the jaw-to-jaw relationship is correct.

- This can be obtained using a lower, plastic, neuromuscular orthotic appliance.

IMPROPER JAW TO JAW RELATIONSHIPS

That cause the condyle to be pushed back

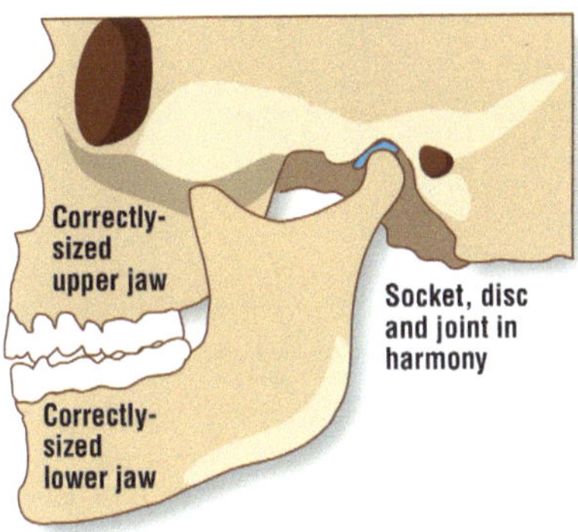

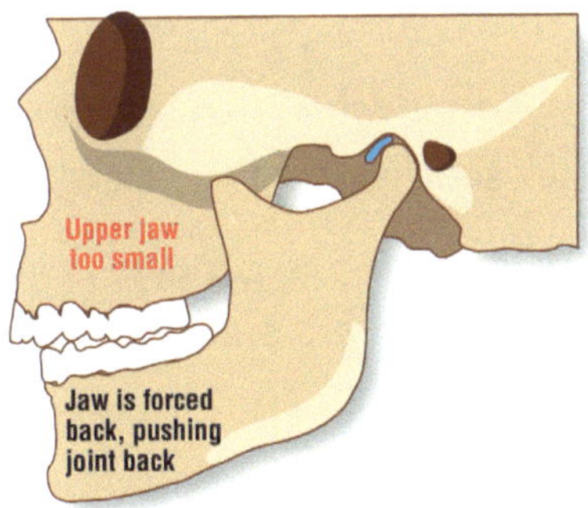

LOWER, REMOVABLE, PLASTIC, NEUROMUSCULAR ORTHOTIC

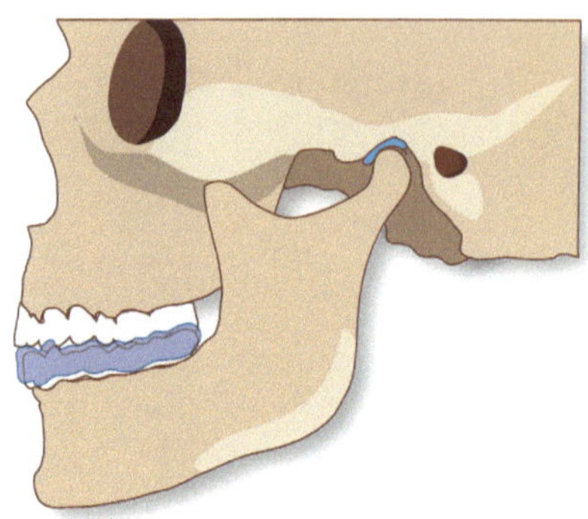

- When the condyle is pushed back too far, it only makes sense to bring it forward.

- Bringing the jaw forward brings the condyle forward.

- When one slides the jaw forward, only the front teeth hit. This can give the joint relief, but one cannot go around with only the front teeth hitting. It is like walking on your toes.

- A neuromuscular orthotic, just like a shoe orthotic, fills in the space of the back teeth when the jaw is forward.

- With the orthotic in place, the condyle is in the proper place and the back teeth are supported as shown in the illustration.

- The neuromuscular orthotic signals the brain that the upper and lower jaw are in harmony!

TREATMENT FOR PAIN IN TM JOINT/EAR AREA

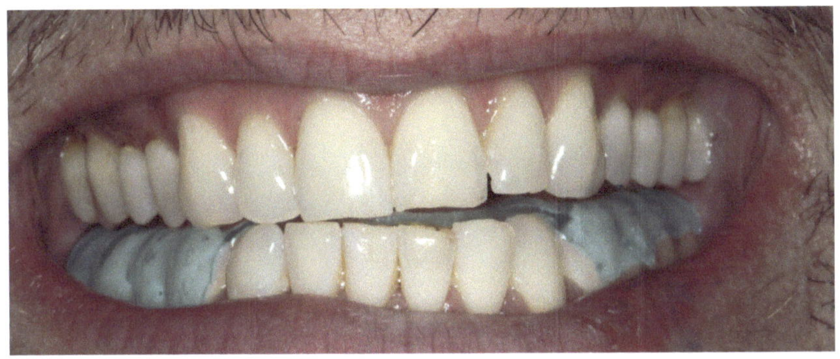

- Look closely at the photo.

- There is a clear, plastic neuromuscular orthotic in between the teeth. (The orthotic of the photo above is colorized blue for the illustration purpose.)

- You can see the upper and lower front teeth are almost end to end, meaning the jaw has been brought forward to the correct upper and lower jaw-to-jaw relationship.

- Looking closer, you can see more space on the left side than the right indicating a torqued mandible.

- When one side of the jaw hits before the other side, it torques the system and the muscles of the head and neck don't like that.

- A torqued mandible fatigues the muscles and can cause muscle pain just like one leg being shorter than the other.

TREATMENT FOR PAIN IN TM JOINT/EAR AREA

PEOPLE WHO SUFFERED FROM TMD PAIN/FOUND RELIEF FROM ORTHOTICS

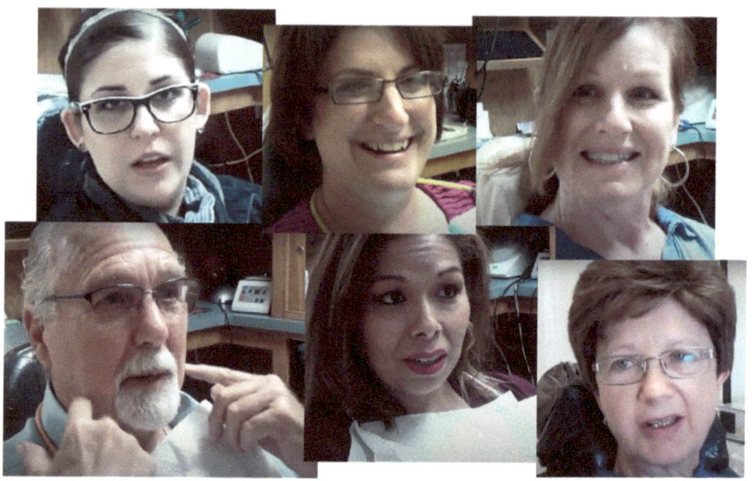

- How painful can myofascial pain be? The answer is mild to life robbing.

- There are as many TMD symptoms as stars in the sky.

  - https://www.youtube.com/watch?v=eojeFP2CxlQ&t=38s

  - https://www.youtube.com/watch?v=wTUyI-zqM3k

  - https://www.youtube.com/watch?v=HnvsdHnpKG0&t=3s

  - https://www.youtube.com/watch?v=nF9G6RQEq74

  - https://www.youtube.com/watch?v=umVcrS1Avzk

TREATMENT FOR PAIN IN TM JOINT/EAR AREA

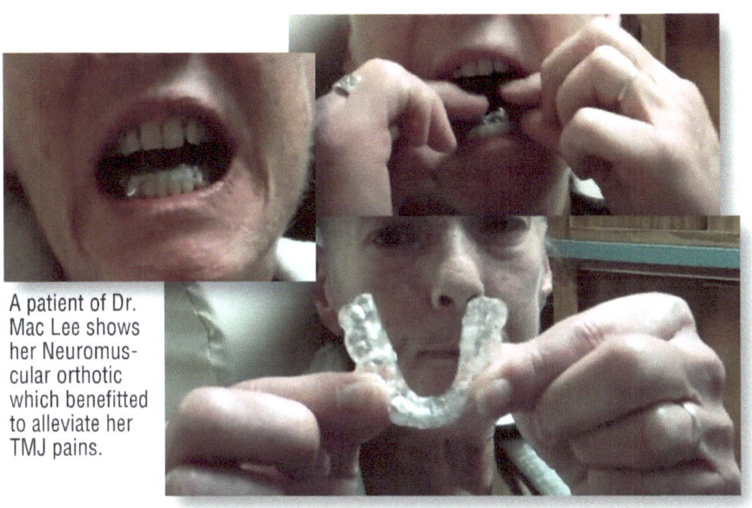

A patient of Dr. Mac Lee shows her Neuromuscular orthotic which benefitted to alleviate her TMJ pains.

- https://www.youtube.com/watch?v=adXWPpYEp5k

- What makes a neuromuscular orthotic different from a look alike plastic splint or night guard is the experience and knowledge of the treating dentist.

- They must know and understand where the lower jaw wants and needs to go to have the proper relationship with the upper jaw.

- Just as important, they need to be able to get that relationship information to the dental lab so a proper TMD orthotic can be made.

CHAPTER SIX: HEADACHES AND OTHER TMD PAINS AND SYMPTOMS

- Headaches

- Migraine like pain

- Trigeminal Neuralgia like pain

- Limited Opening

- Facial pain

- Hot and cold sensitive teeth

- Difficulty in chewing

- Tingling fingertips

- Awakened at night with headache

- Morning headaches

Note: All of the above symptoms may or may not be due to TMD.

HEADACHES AND OTHER TMD PAINS AND SYMPTOMS

- Not all TMD pain is in the ear area.

- TMD pain can be in the temple area, the sides of the face, behind the eyes, in the neck.

- It can create headaches during sleep or upon waking.

- It can create headaches in the daytime especially during emotional times.

- It can make ears feel stuffy.

- In fact, there are more variations of pain due to TMD than stars in the sky.

- This is another reason TMD is confusing to all!

HEADACHES AND OTHER TMD PAINS AND SYMPTOMS

- **Your life robbing pain can be due to muscle spasms in head and neck.**

- You can have horrible head pain with no discomfort in the joint.

- People in pain go to a medical doctor because they think they have a medical condition.

- Since the MD, ENT, neurologist or Nurse Practitioners are often ignorant of TMD, they dismiss you and your pain.

- A well-trained neuromuscular dentist is the first step in stopping the pain.

- The following slides will describe, in layman's terms, why you are in pain and how a neuromuscular dentist can help.

THE HEAD IS A MASS OF MUSCLES, NERVES, TENDONS, LIGAMENTS AND FASCIA

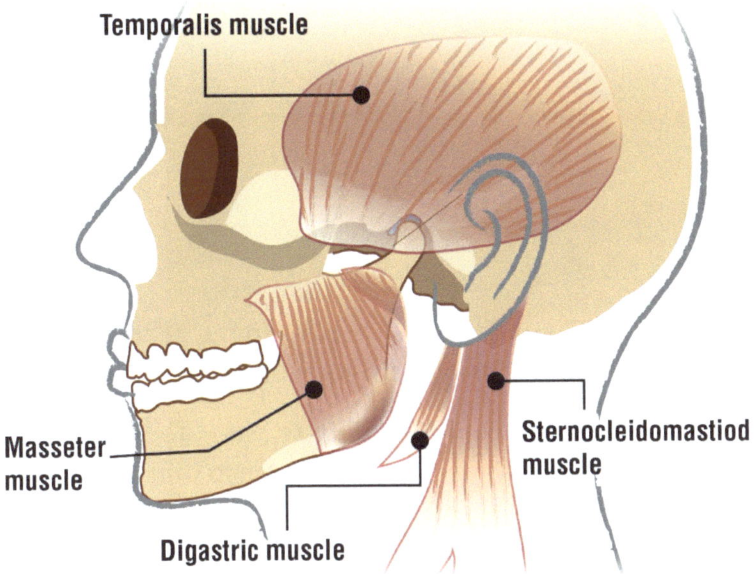

- Put your fingers on your temples and bite down. Feel the muscle movement?

- If you are now having pain in the temple, move your fingers around pressing firmly. Did you find a painful area? Did it feel like a knot.

- Do the same with the jaw muscles.

- And the same with the muscle down the side of the neck.

THE HEAD IS A MASS OF MUSCLES, NERVES, TENDONS, LIGAMENTS AND FASCIA

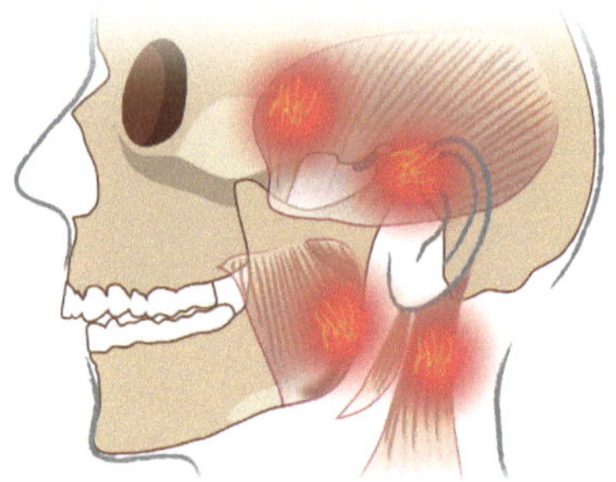

- TMD pain is coming from the muscles in the head. They are being overworked and classified as Myofascial pain.

- *"The most common **causes** of **muscle pain** are tension, stress, overuse and minor injuries."* Mayo Clinic

- *"**Chronic** myofascial **pain** (CMP), also **called** myofascial **pain** syndrome, is a **painful** condition that affects the **muscles** and the sheath of the tissue — **called** the fascia — that surround the **muscles**."* Cleveland Clinic Mar 27, 2019

- **The myofascial pain usually manifests itself via trigger points indicated in the image.**

- **Simply put, the muscles are being overworked while looking for a comfortable home for the jaw to close into.**

THE HEAD IS A MASS OF MUSCLES, NERVES, TENDONS, LIGAMENTS AND FASCIA

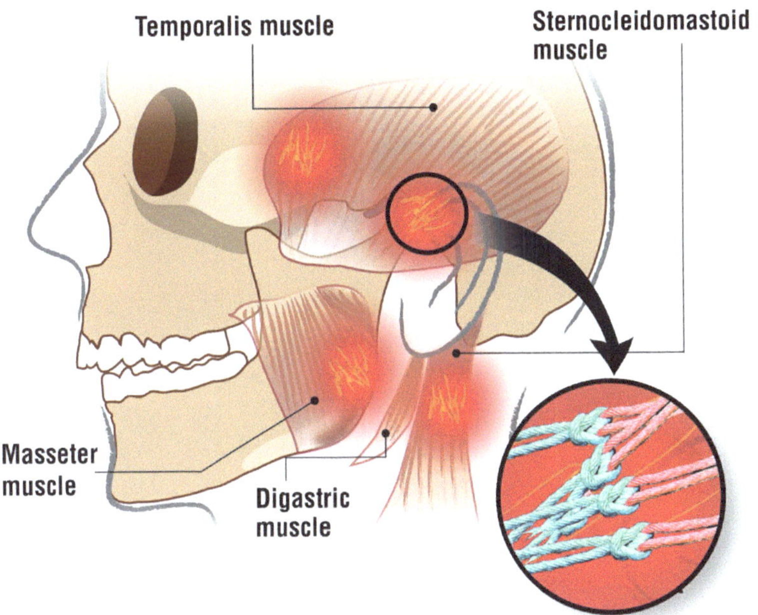

- Trigger points are knots in the muscles as demonstrated in the illustration. Knots just like the cover of this book!

- A properly trained neuromuscular dentist can help with your Myofascial Pain.

- Special Ultra Low Freqency Dental TENS units are used to pulse the muscles of the head and neck, pumping out toxins and relaxing the muscles.

- The TENS unit is either a J5 or QuadraTens which are FDA approved specifically electrical nerve stimulators to relax the muscles of the jaw, head and neck.

- The ULF TENS unit is used prior to and while taking jaw alignment records for a neuromuscular orthotic.

- See example of how an ULF TENS unit relaxes painful muscles of the jaw, head and neck:

https://www.youtube.com/watch?v=5Z0hliSJn-o

https://www.youtube.com/watch?v=gKXvnxoL3k0

CHAPTER SEVEN: TREATMENT FOR TENSION HEADACHES AND MIGRAINES

- Treatment for head, ear, eye and neck pain is a lower, removable, or fixed, plastic neuromuscular orthotic that is basically the same as the one for joint problems.

- The upcoming photograph of a mouth shows patient's jaw is torqued meaning one side hits before the other which creates overworked muscles same as one leg being shorter than the other.

- The neuromuscular orthotic signals the brain that the bite is balanced just as a foot orthotic does.

- Once the TMD orthotic gives you relief there are possible long term treatment options later down the line.

- There are only a small percentage of dentists who are trained in neuromuscular dentistry. If they do not use the ULF TENS, they are not practicing standard NM dentistry.

- There are different treatment philosophies of how to treat TMD other than neuromuscular. I have studied and used most of them with varying degrees of success since 1978. As the author of this book, I have personally found the neurom-uscular principles to be the most predictable for me.

POSSIBLE SELF TREATMENT

- Controlling your TMD pain without the help of a TMD dentist is difficult.

- Stress plays a huge role in TMD as it does in many other health conditions.

- During the day, one can help control TMD by keeping their lips together and teeth apart while placing their tongue in the roof of the mouth, towards the front. This is not easy to do but it helps relax muscles.

- If your TMD is in the ear area, do what ever you can to keep the jaw slightly forward.

- Any stress releasing exercises are important.

- Unfortunately, while sleeping all bets are off on self treatment.

CHAPTER EIGHT: FINDING THE RIGHT DENTIST

- The first step towards healing is understanding your problem which is described in this book.

- The question "Why Me?" is answered by understanding that you have trigger points and other TMD patients may not.

- The next step is finding a dentist trained in neuromuscular dentistry.

- It is imperative that you and the dentist you find have a trusting relationship.

- If you cannot communicate with the treating dentist, the outcome might not be as desired.

- If the dentist is not using an ULF TENS unit, you must ask why and get a satisfactory answer.

- All neuromuscular dentists should take their time to listen to you and understand your pain. This takes time and cannot be rushed.

FINDING THE RIGHT DENTIST

- For a good starting point, go to ICCMO's website search engine at https://iccmo.org/Home/Search to see if there is a member near you.

- All members of ICCMO have had some training in NM dentistry. All members of ICCMO should be using an ULF TENS to relax the jaw muscles.

- Dentists and other health care providers interested in NMD may apply to become members of ICCMO.

- The Executive Board of ICCMO recognized the need to implement a standardized mechanism to assess and insure Neuromuscular competency via Fellowship and Mastership status.

- Those neuromuscular dentists who have obtained their Fellowship or Mastership recognition, have proven to ICCMO that they operate at the highest standards.

- When using the Search Engine, a FICCMO designation designates Fellowship status and MICCMO designates Mastership status.

TM JOINT PAIN SUMMARY

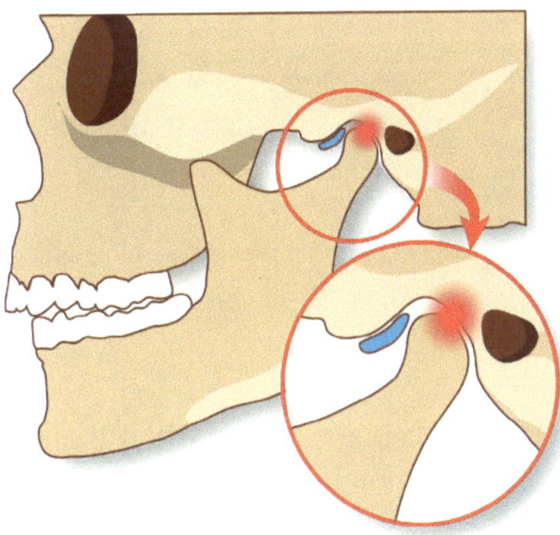

- By now, you have learned that when there is pain in the TM joint itself, odds are that the condlye is too far back pushing against the nerves and vessels behind the condyle as the illustration demonstrates.

- Your dentist needs to know how to make you a lower, plastic neuromuscular orthotic that allows the jaw to come forward bringing the condyle forward and away from the nerves.

- Neuromuscular trained dentists, using special knowledge and equipment, know how to make such an appliance.

- ICCMO.org is the original Neuromuscular organization and the first place to start your research.

LIFE ROBBING PAIN SUMMARY

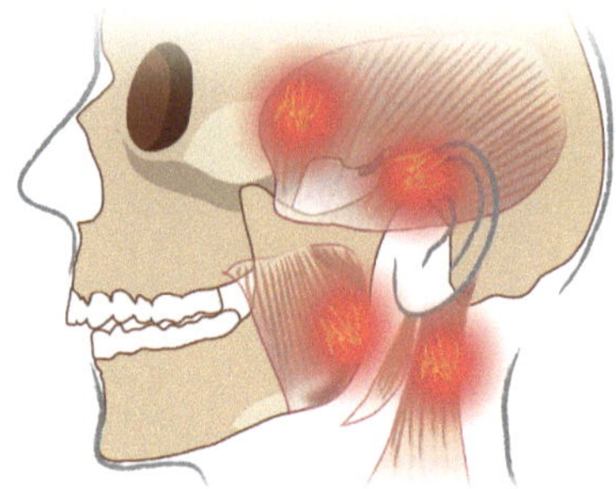

- By now, you have also learned that when there is life robbing pain in the head and neck, as the illustration demonstrates, the pain is often due to trigger points in the muscles.

- The trigger points are due to over worked, fatiqued muscles compensating for an improper jaw-to-jaw relationship.

- Your dentist needs to know how to make you a lower, plastic neuromuscular orthotic that allows the jaw to close in the correct orthopedic position which relaxes the muscles.

- Neuromuscular trained dentists, using special knowledge and equipment, know how to make such an appliance.

- ICCMO.org is the original Neuromuscular organization and the first place to start your research.

A MESSAGE FROM THE BOARD OF REGENTS OF ICCMO

- ICCMO was created to help dentists serve TMD pain patients looking for answers.

- What you have learned in this book is not taught in most dental schools and therefore few dentists are trained in properly treating patients suffering from TMD pain.

- If you have a good relationship with your dentist, please share this information. ICCMO will be able to help train your dentist on how to help you.

- If there are no ICCMO dentists in your area, search for a Neuromuscular Dentist. If you find one you like, share this information so he or she will join ICCMO and then can be found on its search engine.

- Good luck in your search and know your pain is real and there is help for your specific needs.

Disclaimer

This ebook is intended to provide information and not dental or medical advice. An appropriate diagnosis and treatment plan for any patient can be made only by a treating dentist, physician, or group of doctors. ICCMO nor the author, Dr. Mac Lee, shall have no liability or responsibility to any person with respect to loss or damage caused or alleged to be caused directly or indirectly by the information contained in this e-book or obtained from other websites to which a visitor may connect and view.

Author: Dr. Mac Lee

Cover art by: Kimiko Peterson.

9 7 9 8 7 0 2 0 6 8 3 3 6